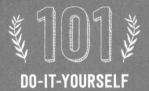

101

DO-IT-YOURSELF

FACE
MASKS

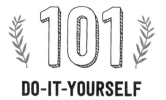

101

DO-IT-YOURSELF

FACE
MASKS

FUN, HEALTHY, ALL-NATURAL
SHEET MASKS FOR EVERY SKIN TYPE

JENNIFER McCARTNEY

The Countryman Press
A division of W. W. Norton & Company
Independent Publishers Since 1923

Disclaimer

Some people may be allergic to some of the ingredients used to make these masks. Consult your doctor if you suspect that you may be allergic to any ingredient. Test each mask on a small patch of skin before you apply it to your entire face. Read the descriptions of the different ingredients to be sure that you know which ones may cause adverse skin reactions even if you are not allergic to them. Consult your doctor before using any of these masks if you are currently using any skin medication to make sure that the combination of that medication and the ingredients in the masks will not injure your skin. Consult your doctor if you have a bad skin reaction to any mask. Before letting children make and use any of these masks, make sure that none of them is known to be allergic to the ingredients.

Image Credits

CONTENTS

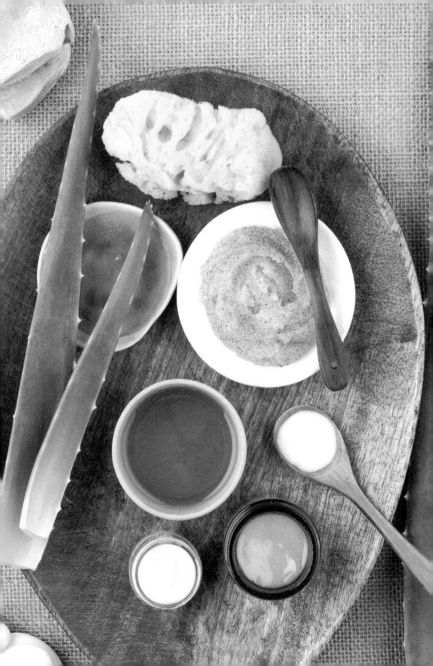

INTRODUCTION
WELCOME TO THE WORLD OF FACE MASKING.
WE'RE GLAD YOU'RE HERE.

*"Nature gives you the face you have
at twenty; it is up to you to merit the
face you have at fifty."*
– Coco Chanel

101 DIY Face Masks is a fun, easy-to-follow guide for creating amazing face masks in the comfort of your own home. The book will teach you how to make your own cotton sheet masks and infuse them with proven homeopathic ingredients found in your kitchen cupboards. You'll also find recipes for traditional masks that get applied straight to your skin, specialty masks for special occasions, and even masks for your lips and hair.

Save money while knowing exactly what you're putting on your face! No more parabens or unpronounceable chemicals! Instead, enjoy the beneficial effects of ingredients like honey, milk, avocado, egg whites, rose water, aloe vera, and even pumpkin. Learn the benefits of each ingredient and how it works—then get to work mixing and masking. With color photos and step-by-step instructions, it's an easy way to have fun and keep your skin healthy without breaking the bank.

Each mask does something awesome for your skin—hydrating, brightening, antiaging, tightening, calming, etc.—and so the recipes in each chapter are organized by that primary benefit. You'll find mask ideas for all ages and skin issues!

SOOTHING & SOFTENING Irritated, angry skin? Then the Bee Calm Honey + Tea Mask is a must-try (page 30).

BRIGHTENING & REFRESHING Dull, oily skin? You need a Brighten-My-Day Lemon Control Mask (page 43).

HEALING & ANTIAGING Dry and peeling winter skin? You definitely need a Coconut Glam Glow Mask (page 46).

WHAT IS A SHEET MASK? A sheet mask is simply a piece of cotton or other material that is shaped to the face and infused with beautifying ingredients. While traditional masks are applied directly to the face and must therefore be thick enough to stick to the skin, a sheet mask can use lighter, more liquid ingredients.

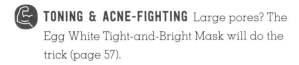

TONING & ACNE-FIGHTING Large pores? The Egg White Tight-and-Bright Mask will do the trick (page 57).

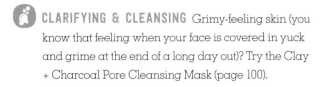

CLARIFYING & CLEANSING Grimy-feeling skin (you know that feeling when your face is covered in yuck and grime at the end of a long day out)? Try the Clay + Charcoal Pore Cleansing Mask (page 100).

HYDRATING & NOURISHING Hungover and dehydrated skin? Try the Charcoal + Aloe Detox-So-I-Can-Retox Mask (page 106).

- - - - - - - - - - - - - -
DIY masks make the perfect slumber party activity. They're fun for all ages—a kid's birthday party or your next bachelorette party. Just don't forget to snap a selfie!
- - - - - - - - - - - - - -

Of course, everyone's skin has different needs, sensitivities, and preferences. Play around and have fun until you find what works for you. Remember skincare is a great opportunity for self-care. So slather on a mask, curl up with a good book, and enjoy your "me time"!

HANDY TOOLS FOR MASKING

The only things you need to make great masks are easy to find and super affordable. You probably already own most, if not all, of them!

- small aluminum or glass bowl for mixing
- hair dye brush for applying traditional masks (optional)
- cotton sheet mask (see page 28 for instructions on making your own)
- washcloth
- fork for mashing
- spoon for mixing
- zipper sandwich bag or small jar with screw-top lid for storing extra mask liquid

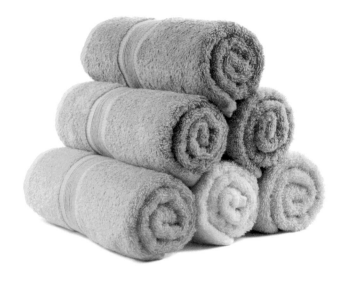

COMMON INGREDIENTS AND THEIR USES

"Invest in your skin. It is going to represent you for a very long time."

—Linden Tyler

Most of the face masks in this book can be made with common ingredients found in your fridge or pantry. A few ingredients, like activated charcoal or aloe vera gel, may or may not already be in one of your cupboards, but they can be easily found at your local health food store or online. The common denominator of all the ingredients is that they're affordable. That means it's easy to experiment with different recipes to find what truly works best for your skin.

Activated Charcoal

Although activated charcoal is a trendy skin-care ingredient now, there are limited studies about the benefits of charcoal for cleansing or detoxing skin. Its main known medical benefits are related to oral consumption and not topical use. But it is thought that with topical use, the charcoal draws out impurities from the skin—making it a great ingredient if you want to reduce the appearance of pores and get rid of black-heads.

Aloe Vera

Aloe vera, which can be found as a topical gel at any drugstore, is packed with beneficial ingredients including vitamins A, B12, C, and E, as well as folic acid, amino acids, and fatty acids. It speeds wound healing, aids in the development of collagen, softens skin, and acts as an antiseptic, making it great for antiaging and problem skin. Fun fact: the word *aloe* derives from the Arabic word "Alloeh," which means "shining bitter substance."

Apple Cider Vinegar

Apple cider vinegar is antibacterial and antifungal. It contains malic acid, a potent alpha hydroxy acid (AHA), which makes it a great toner for smoothing and softening skin. It is also good for oily skin. Be sure to dilute with water before using directly on the skin, and use no more than once a week.

Avocado

There is some evidence that topical application of avocados can help protect the skin against UV rays by penetrating skin cells to destroy free radicals associated with UV damage. It's also rich in vitamins C, D, and E, as well as being an excellent moisturizer. (Eating avocados has also been shown to increase collagen levels in skin. So use one half of the fruit on your face and eat the other half for double the results!) Excellent for dry or aging skin.

Baking Soda

Baking soda has long been used as a natural exfoliator, although it should be used sparingly and is not for sensitive skin. Baking soda has a high pH level of 9, while our skin has a normal pH of about 4.5. Use it too frequently and you can disrupt your skin's natural acidity. For some skincare lovers, however, baking soda is a holy grail that helps control acne and oil while exfoliating and brightening the skin.

Banana

Bananas contain potassium as well as natural oils that make it a great moisturizer. The banana fruit has also been found to have antibacterial and antifungal properties that make it useful for treating acne and skin inflammation.

Brown Sugar

Brown sugar is a wonderful (and affordable!) exfoliator for face and lips as long as you're gentle as you apply it. Plus it smells amazing! Use no more than once a week, especially if you have sensitive skin.

Chamomile

Dried chamomile (in other words, chamomile tea) is an antimicrobial, anti-inflammatory, and antioxidant. It's even been approved in Germany for use in wound and burn therapy because of its calming and anti-inflammatory benefits. It's also been proven to diminish signs of UV damage and to improve skin texture and elasticity.

Bentonite Clay

This mineral-rich, oil-absorbing clay has proven to speed wound healing and to absorb excess sebum (the overproduction of which can cause acne). This makes it great for the healing of acne and acne scarring. Fun fact: bentonite clay gets its name from Fort Benton, Wyoming, where the clay is sourced.

French Green Clay

French green clay gets its color from decomposed plant matter such as seaweed. This clay acts to draw out impurities from pores and is packed with minerals like magnesium, calcium, potassium, manganese, phosphorus, silicon, copper, and selenium. It's great for oily skin.

French Pink Clay

A combination of red and white clay, French pink clay is generally thought to be the gentlest of the clays, making it perfect for sensitive skin.

Cocoa Powder

Cocoa powder is an antioxidant that has been shown to improve skin elasticity and positively affect collagen production when applied topically. When ingested, antioxidant flavonols in the cocoa have been proven to limit UV-induced skin damage. It's thought that topical application can have the same effect. Many health and beauty devotees also swear by cacao powder—which is just like cocoa powder except it's unprocessed and raw. You likely already have cocoa powder in the kitchen, but if you want to splurge you can find the higher-end cacao at your local health food store.

Coconut Oil

Antibacterial, antifungal, and extra moisturizing, coconut oil is a great all-purpose skincare ingredient, especially for dry skin. Plus, it smells great!

Coffee Grounds

Coffee has been found to reduce inflammation, redness, and irritation when applied to the skin. The caffeine works to constrict blood vessels, providing temporary relief from these skin concerns. It's also been found to reduce the appearance of cellulite. This is a great ingredient to consider if you're looking to recover from a long flight or a bad hangover that's left your skin feeling bloated, puffy, and dehydrated. Use very finely ground coffee, as it's the gentlest on your skin.

Egg Whites

Egg whites (the part of the raw egg that isn't the yolk) contain both collagen and protein, which can help give skin a plumper appearance. Egg whites can also have a tightening and toning effect.

Honey

While mostly sugar and water, honey is full of amino acids, vitamins, and minerals and has been used as an antimicrobial agent for thousands of years. Medical studies have found that honey can inhibit approximately 60 species of bacteria as well as fungi and even viruses. It also has anti-inflammatory properties and can help heal wounds, making it perfect for common skin issues like acne or psoriasis.

Kiwi

The kiwi is the national fruit of China and has been consumed there since at least the 12th century. Nowadays it's easy to get at any grocery store, which is good news for your skin as the flesh of the kiwifruit is rich in vitamins C, E, and K, and it acts as an exfoliant. It's also a known allergen, so be sure to do a skin patch test before using it on your face, or avoid it completely if you already know you're allergic.

Lemon Juice

Lemon juice is useful for brightening and evening out skin tone as well as fighting hyperpigmentation such as acne scars or age spots. It works as a natural exfoliator and antibacterial agent as well. Lemon juice can cause photosensitivity though, so be sure to use it sparingly and limit your skin's sun exposure after using it.

Matcha Green Tea Powder

Green tea isn't just for drinking anymore. Topical application has been proven to provide lasting protection against UV damage as well as to reduce DNA damage sustained after sun exposure. This is thought to be because of the polyphenols contained in the tea, which have anti-inflammatory and anticarcinogenic properties. Matcha has more antioxidants than regular green tea, so it's a great one to use in skincare. If you don't have matcha, then regular green tea will suffice.

Milk

Milk has been used in skincare routines for centuries because of its moisturizing, calming, and exfoliating properties. This is due to the lactic acid (an AHA) contained within. Both Cleopatra and Queen Elizabeth enjoyed bathing in milk. While these monarchs likely luxuriated in goat or donkey milk, regular cow milk or powdered milk works just as well for today's modern woman. If you have extra dry skin, try using yogurt instead for an even more moisturizing effect.

Oatmeal

Oatmeal has been clinically proven to reduce dryness, itching, scaling, and roughness when applied topically. In fact, oatmeal is FDA-approved for treating minor skin irritation. A classic home skincare remedy, it's been used to treat dermatological issues for centuries going back to Roman times. For skincare, it's best to use colloidal oatmeal, which is whole oats that have been finely milled and therefore are more easily absorbed by the skin.

Pineapple Juice

Packed with vitamin C and antioxidants, pineapple juice also contains the enzyme bromelain that is thought to soften the skin, reduce inflammation, and target the appearance of fine lines, acne, and sun-damaged skin.

Pumpkin

Pumpkin is having a comeback moment. Lots of big skincare brands are debuting product lines with pumpkin as the main ingredient—and with good reason. Pumpkin has a ton of fruit enzymes and alpha hydroxy acids as well as vitamins A and C. That means pumpkin masks can help exfoliate and brighten skin at the cellular level as well as boost collagen production, making it perfect for damaged or aging skin.

Rice Flour

Rice flour (also called *rice bran* or *rice powder*) is exactly what it sounds like—grains of rice that have been finely ground into a flour. It has been used for centuries in places like Japan to target hyperpigmentation and to brighten dull or aging skin. The flour has oil-absorbing properties that make it a good choice for oily skin, and it also acts as a light mechanical exfoliant. It contains ferulic acid, which is thought to provide antioxidant benefits as well.

Rose Hip Seed Oil

There are lots of face oils on the market that are good for your skin—from argan oil to hempseed oil. If you've already got a favorite face oil then feel free to substitute that into the face mask recipes calling for rose hip seed oil. Rose hip seed oil is a light, affordable, and versatile oil rich in vitamin A and linoleic acid. It works as a moisturizer, reduces skin damage and signs of photoaging, and lessens scars and imperfections. Harvested from (you guessed it) seeds from the rosebush, rose hip seed oil is available online or at most health and beauty stores. It should be refrigerated.

Rose Water

Rose water is made from exactly what it sounds like: water and rose petals. It's been used in skincare (and in the kitchen!) for centuries in places such as Iran and Syria. It has antioxidant and anti-inflammatory properties, and of course it smells wonderful. Rose scent is thought to have a calming effect on the central nervous system. Rose water is available for purchase online or at specialty health and beauty stores.

Seaweed

Seaweed is jam-packed with vitamins A and C as well as minerals like potassium, iron, iodine, and magnesium. It's also antibacterial, anti-inflammatory, and very hydrating. Because of seaweed's many benefits you'll find it listed as an ingredient in various high-end beauty products! For aging skin and healing acne, this is a must-try ingredient.

Turmeric

There is scientific evidence that topical applications of turmeric can improve skin health. Curcumin, an active component in turmeric, has both antimicrobial and antioxidant properties. It also may provide lasting protection against UV damage. It is terrific for acne-prone skin or skin that needs detoxing and calming.

Be careful though—turmeric is strongly pigmented and can stain your clothes, counters, and towels. For any recipe that requires turmeric, I suggest doing a test patch on your skin to ensure it doesn't result in discoloration. Baking soda and lemon juice can remove turmeric stains from your skin and countertops. Coconut oil will also remove turmeric staining from the skin—just apply a few drops of oil to a cotton ball and wipe over skin. To further guard against staining, be sure to use old or dark towels and a stainless steel bowl for mixing.

Watermelon

Watermelon is rich in lycopene, lactic acid, and vitamins A, B6, and C. As watermelon is about 90 percent water, it absorbs well into the skin and is a perfect light moisturizer.

Yogurt

Yogurt can help improve the moisture, brightness, and elasticity of skin. The lactic acid in yogurt can help dissolve dead skin cells and tighten pores, while the active cultures can help with acne, eczema, or problem skin. It is also great for dry skin. Try to use natural yogurt brands with no added sugar—plain Greek yogurt is an ideal option.

NOTE ON ESSENTIAL OILS   Essential oils like lavender and tea tree have been used for centuries in skincare. They smell great and have many healing properties. They can also, unfortunately, occasionally be skin irritants for sensitive skin, which is why I've avoided including them in most of the following recipes. But if you know your skin can handle them (and you've done a skin patch test), feel free to add a drop or two of essential oil to any of these masks according to your skin needs! Just be sure to avoid using the mask near the eye area.

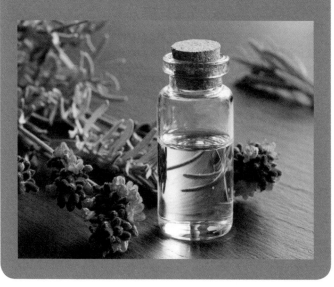

A PRIMER ON ACIDS

Incorporating acids into your skincare is very important, especially as your skin ages and experiences photodamage from the sun. But what are acids exactly? Acids are a class of chemical compounds that come in many forms. They occur naturally in everything from milk to sugarcane. When applied to skin, an acid acts as a chemical exfoliator, removing the top layer of dead surface skin, which in turn reduces the appearance of wrinkles by smoothing fine lines and improves skin tone and texture. The most common type of acid group is the alpha hydroxy acids (AHAs). Ingredients like milk and yogurt (high in lactic acid), apple cider vinegar (malic acid), and lemon (citric acid), all contain AHAs. For the purposes of this book we'll be dealing mainly with lactic, malic, and citric acids as they are found in common household ingredients. Common AHAs found in store-bought skincare products include glycolic and salicylic acids. These are not typically found in natural ingredients, with the notable exception of pineapple, which contains glycolic acid.

COMMON AHAs

Lactic Acid

A gentle exfoliating and moisturizing acid derived from milk.

Citric Acid

A mild AHA found in in the flesh and juice of citrus fruits.

Malic Acid

A mild AHA derived from apples.

Glycolic Acid

A strong exfoliating acid derived from sugarcane and also found in pineapples.

Salicylic Acid

A strong, made-in-the-laboratory acid found mostly in store-bought products.

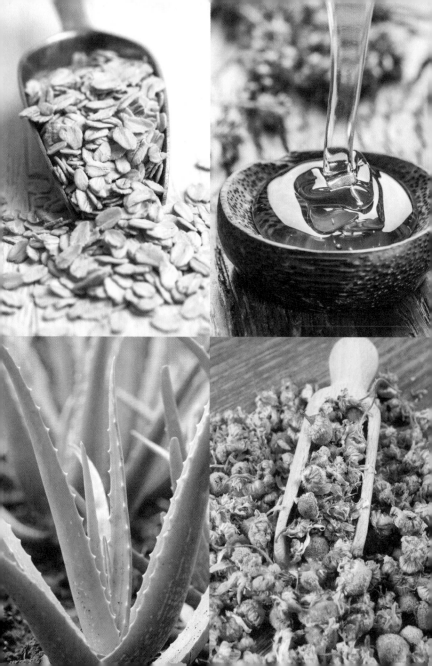

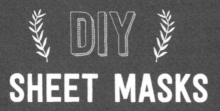

DIY
SHEET MASKS

"You're never too old to become younger."
– Mae West

Single-use cotton masks infused with beautifying essences have become a skincare staple thanks to the popularity and high quality of Korean beauty products (sheet masking originated in Korea). Sephora alone carries more than 100 different types of masks by brands both big and small. Celebrities are sheet masking too! Everyone from Bella Hadid and Katy Perry to Goldie Hawn and Neil Patrick Harris has posted a selfie wearing a sheet mask. With their selfie-friendly style and ease of use, it's no wonder sheet masking has taken off. Not only are the masks easy to use (no mess on your hands or in your sink), they also allow the ingredients to be absorbed directly into your skin without evaporating or drying out—genius!

MAKE YOUR OWN BESPOKE, REUSABLE COTTON SHEET MASK

Affordability and sustainability are both great reasons for DIY sheet masking. Why waste your money on a five-dollar mask you can only use once, when you can make your own reusable cloth face mask (washer- and dryer-friendly) and create dozens of your own homemade, all-natural masks for every skin concern? Single-use, store-bought masks are also bad for the environment—who wants to trash a whole sheet of cotton and its plastic packaging every time you hydrate your skin? So the first step to great skin? Make your own mask!

Buy a set of cotton cloths online or at your local fabric store (natural, undyed muslin works best as it's light and breathable and will hold the mask ingredients well). This should cost you about five dollars. Cut the cloth into a circle that fits your face without overlapping your hairline. Then cut holes for your eyes, nostrils, and mouth. To help the mask fit snugly to your face without bunching, cut two small slits about an inch long on either side of where the sheet covers your chin (horizontal or vertical slits both work). If you like, you can use an existing single-use face mask* as a guide or find a template online.

* *

*Don't reuse a single-use, store-bought mask with your own mask liquids. You can't be sure what a store-bought mask is made of or which chemicals or substances remain in the material. Also, you won't be able to throw it in the washing machine like a pure cotton mask, and the combination of whatever substances have already been absorbed in the mask with the ingredients you're using could cause skin irritation.

* *

A NOTE ON SHEET MASKS VERSUS TRADITIONAL FACE MASKS Sheet masks work well with light, easy-to-absorb ingredients that will saturate and penetrate the cotton mask, such as egg whites, watermelon, herbal teas, and aloe vera. Thicker ingredients like mashed avocado, yogurt, and banana work better applied directly to the face.

Using and Reusing Your Bespoke Sheet Mask

Sheet masks are very simple to use. Simply soak a mask in the liquid of your choice. Then place it on that gorgeous face of yours and leave there for the prescribed amount of time in the mask recipe.

After you use the mask, just toss it in the washer, or handwash it if you prefer, using a gentle, unscented laundry detergent—the more natural, the better. You can then hang the mask out to dry or throw it in the dryer, sans dryer sheet.

Pop a single-use mask soaked in your treatment of choice into a zipper sandwich bag and take it with you when you travel.

Give the Gift of Sheet Masking

A DIY sheet mask makes a great gift. Layer a few cloth masks in a reusable jar and fill with your favorite skin-saving treatment. Add a tag that lists the ingredients and instructions, and maybe a ribbon or two. Voilà!

SOOTHING & SOFTENING

SHEET MASKS

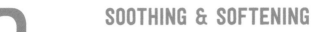

THE BEE CALM HONEY + TEA MASK

---

2 tablespoons honey
¼ cup chamomile tea, cooled
1 teaspoon lemon juice

Honey is a great antibacterial treatment while the chamomile works to soothe skin and calm breakouts or dryness. The lemon works as a brightening agent. Zap the honey in the microwave for 10 seconds to warm it up. Combine with the cooled chamomile tea and lemon juice. Soak a dry sheet mask in the liquid and apply to face. Leave on for 15 minutes, then wash face as usual.

. . . .

Lemon juice can cause photosensitivity, so be sure to use it sparingly and to limit your skin's sun exposure after using it.

. . . .

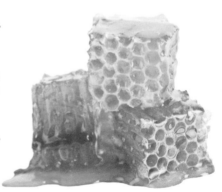

WATERMELON + ALOE FRESH-FACED MASK

2 tablespoons aloe vera gel
¼ cup watermelon juice

The soothing and healing properties of aloe vera combine with the light brightening and moisturizing properties of watermelon in this mask that's perfect for sunburned summer skin. Combine ingredients and soak a dry sheet mask in the liquid. Apply mask to face and let sit for 15 minutes. Remove cotton mask and pat the remaining liquid into the skin.

CHAMOMILE + ROSE WATER MASK

2 tablespoons chamomile tea, cooled
1 tablespoon rose water

Soothe and hydrate skin as well as reduce inflammation with this chamomile and rose mask. Combine the two ingredients and soak a dry sheet mask in the liquid. Place on face for 15 minutes, then remove, patting excess liquid into skin.

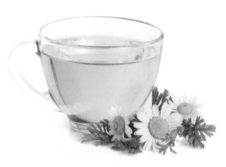

PINEAPPLE PEEL MASK

2 tablespoons pineapple juice

Let the skin-softening properties of the pineapple's bromelain enzyme work their magic for you. Soak the dry sheet mask in the pineapple juice and apply to face. Let sit for 15 minutes, then remove mask and pat remaining liquid into the skin.

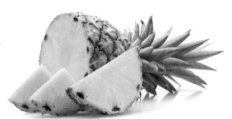

HONEY + MILK FACIAL MASK

2 tablespoons whole milk
1 tablespoon honey

Milk and honey are a classic combination that's been used in skincare for centuries. Classic, effective, and simple, this milk and honey mask will leave your skin feeling soft and supple. Combine the two ingredients. Soak the dry sheet mask in the liquid and apply to face. Leave on for 15 minutes, then remove and pat remaining liquid into skin.

"I'm a big believer in that if you focus on good skincare . . . you really won't need a lot of makeup."

– Demi Moore

BALANCE MATCHA MASK

1 tablespoon matcha powder
1 tablespoon coconut oil, warmed
1 tablespoon chamomile tea, cooled
1 teaspoon honey

Find balance with this calming matcha powder sheet mask. Combine ingredients and dip sheet mask in liquid. Place mask on face and leave on for 15 minutes. Remove mask, then rinse face with warm water.

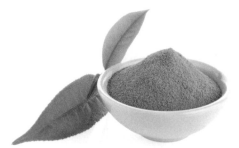

You can use finely ground green tea if you don't have matcha on hand.

COCONUT OIL DEEP CONDITIONING HAIR MOISTURE MASK

¼ cup coconut oil, warmed
1 ripe banana, mashed
1 tablespoon honey

Coconut oil is a fantastic, low-cost healthy hair essential. The natural oil will bring shine and vitality to most hair types. Mix the ingredients together to form a paste. Using your hands or a hair dye brush, apply the mask evenly throughout dry hair, starting at the roots and working your way to the ends. Leave the mask on for 30 minutes. Wash thoroughly with a gentle shampoo but don't use conditioner.

Depending on the length and thickness of your hair, there may be some mask left over. Pop it into a resealable plastic bag or jar and store in the fridge. It will keep for about a week.

If you have longer or thicker hair, you may need to increase the amount of coconut oil. For those with thin or very short hair, the oil can be a bit heavy and you may want to use less or omit altogether.

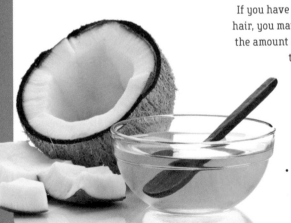

CALMING CHAMOMILE + OATMEAL MASK

1 tablespoon colloidal oatmeal
¼ cup chamomile tea, cooled
1 tablespoon whole milk

Oatmeal soothes and calms irritated skin and the same is true of chamomile tea. This double whammy calming mask is perfect for use ahead of special events (graduations, bridal showers, etc.) where you want soothed, calm skin—save the chemical peels and irritating ingredients for another day. Plus, the light exfoliating properties of the milky lactic acid and oatmeal give you an extra boost of gentle cleansing.

Mix the oatmeal in the chamomile tea and milk until dissolved. Soak a clean dry cotton sheet mask in the liquid and apply to face. Let dry for 15 minutes, then gently rinse face with warm water.

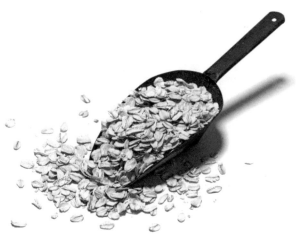

ROSE WATER + HONEY NOURISH-AND-REPAIR MASK

2 tablespoons rose water
1 tablespoon honey
1 tablespoon aloe vera gel

Gentle rose water penetrates the skin to soothe irritation, while honey and aloe hydrate and protect. Combine the ingredients. Dip the sheet mask into the liquid and apply to face, letting the calming scent of the rose and honey relax you. Leave on for 15 minutes, then gently wash off with warm water.

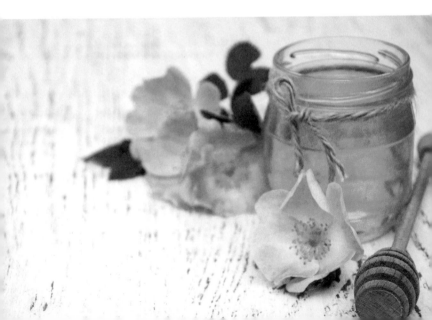

HYDRATING & NOURISHING
SHEET MASKS

BUTTERMILK LACTIC ACID MASK

2 tablespoons buttermilk

Buttermilk is a gentle, moisturizing, pH-balanced mask that will leave your skin refreshed and renewed thanks to the lactic acid. Soak a dry sheet mask in the buttermilk and apply to face. Leave on for 15 minutes, then remove and pat remaining fluid into skin.

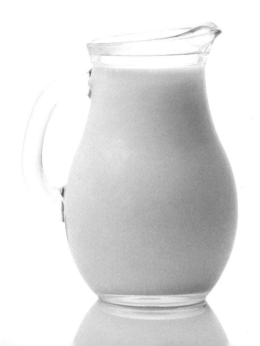

MATCHA + SEAWEED MASK

¼ cup brewed matcha tea, cooled
1 package of dried seaweed

Okay, so not everyone has seaweed lying around, but it's easy to find at most grocery stores or online. It comes in dried strips, which are perfect for sheet masking—no cotton mask needed! Plus the minerals (iron and calcium) and vitamins (A and C) found in the seaweed pack a powerful punch for your skin. Brew a strong matcha tea and let cool. Dip the seaweed strips into the matcha tea and then lay them on your face and neck until covered. Leave on for 15 minutes and remove the strips, patting any excess fluid into the skin.

Make sure you get seaweed that doesn't have any additional ingredients, such as salt. You can use finely ground green tea if you don't have matcha on hand.

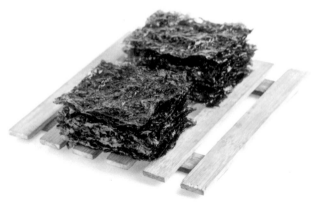

ALOE NOURISH-AND-REVITALIZE MASK

2 tablespoons aloe vera gel
2 seaweed strips, crushed into flakes
1 teaspoon coconut oil, warmed

Soothing aloe vera with mineral-enriched seaweed make a plant-based mask that will hydrate while plumping and repairing skin. Mix the aloe, seaweed flakes, and coconut oil together until combined. Dip the mask into the liquid and apply to face. Leave on for 15 minutes, then remove mask, rinsing face with warm water.

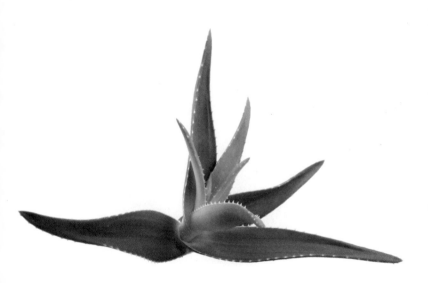

HYDRATION BOOST MASK

1 tablespoon watermelon juice
1 teaspoon aloe vera gel
1 teaspoon honey
1 teaspoon rose water

Why use one powerful hydration tool when you can use a bunch! This all-purpose moisture mask provides intense moisture without feeling heavy or oily. Combine the watermelon juice, aloe, honey, and rose water. Soak a dry sheet mask in the liquid. Apply to face and leave on for 15 minutes. Remove mask and pat remaining liquid into skin.

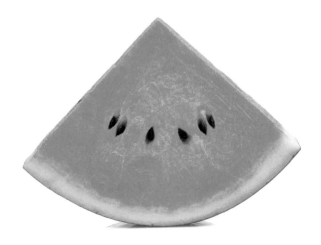

BRIGHTENING & REFRESHING
SHEET MASKS

VITAMIN C REPAIR MASK

---

2 teaspoons lime juice

2 teaspoons lemon juice

2 teaspoons pineapple juice

2 teaspoons grapefruit juice

2 teaspoons aloe vera gel

For brightening skin while reducing scarring and pigmentation, you can't go wrong with the damaged-skin-zapping power of vitamin C. Combine the fruit juices together with the aloe. Dip a dry sheet mask into the liquid and apply to face. Leave on for 15 minutes, remove mask, and pat remaining liquid into skin.

• • • • • • • • • • • • • • •

Lemon juice can cause photosensitivity, so be sure to use it sparingly and to limit your skin's sun exposure after using it.

• • • • • • • • • • • • • • •

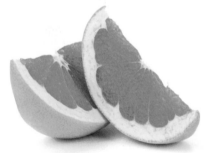

ROSE HIP + COCONUT LUSH LOVE MASK

1 teaspoon rose hip seed oil
1 tablespoon coconut oil, warmed
1 tablespoon aloe vera gel

For hydrating repair there's no better combo than rose hip seed oil and coconut oil. Both oils are antibacterial, nourishing, and moisturizing—you'll be left with smooth, soft, and hydrated skin. Combine the rose hip seed oil, coconut oil, and aloe. Dip a dry sheet mask in the liquid and apply to face. Let sit for 15 minutes and remove the mask, patting any remaining liquid into the skin.

You can substitute any of your favorite face oils for rose hip seed oil.

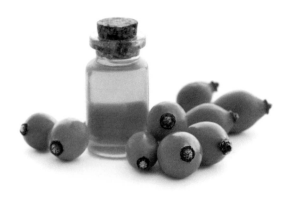

BRIGHTEN-MY-DAY LEMON CONTROL MASK

2 tablespoons lemon juice
1 egg white

Allow the properties of lemon to brighten skin and cut through oil, while the egg white tightens and firms. Combine the lemon juice and egg white and then soak the dry sheet mask in the liquid. Apply to face and leave on for 15 minutes. Rinse face gently with warm water.

. . . .

Lemon juice can cause photosensitivity, so be sure to use it sparingly and to limit your skin's sun exposure after using it.

. . . .

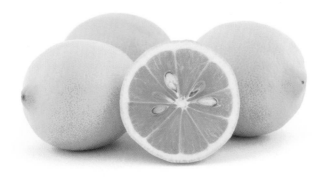

WATERMELON + PINEAPPLE FRUIT MASK

2 tablespoons pineapple juice
¼ cup watermelon juice

Pineapple's hardworking glycolic acid will dissolve old skin cells and reveal fresh skin underneath, while the watermelon will hydrate and brighten. Combine the pineapple and watermelon juice and then soak a dry sheet mask in the liquid. Apply sheet mask to face (warning: it will smell amazing) and let sit for 15 minutes. Remove mask and pat any excess fluid into the skin.

SUMMER WATERMELON + HONEY MASK

¼ cup watermelon juice
1 tablespoon honey

This is a light, refreshing mask that's perfect for summer and for all skin types. The watermelon serves to brighten, hydrate, and freshen the skin, while the honey acts as a natural moisturizer. Soak a dry sheet mask in the liquid and apply to face (this one will definitely drip so be careful!). Leave on for 15 minutes, then wash face as usual or pat remaining liquid into skin.

SWEET SUGAR EXFOLIATING LIP SCRUB AND MASK

1 teaspoon brown sugar
1 teaspoon coconut oil, warmed

Talk about delicious! This scrub and moisturizing lip mask isn't for eating—although it's 100-percent natural and nontoxic. Mix the ingredients together to form a paste. Rub the scrub gently into your lips for about 10 seconds. Then leave the lip mask on for 5–10 minutes. Gently rinse off the lip mask.

Brown sugar should be used no more than once a week, especially if you have sensitive skin.

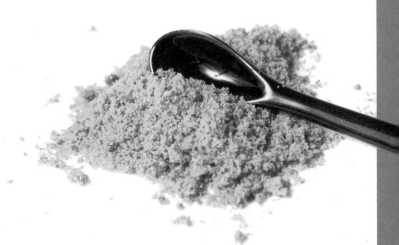

HEALING & ANTIAGING

SHEET MASKS

COCONUT GLAM GLOW MASK

2 tablespoons coconut oil, warmed
1 teaspoon honey

This mask is a must-have balm for dull and dry skin needing the restorative power of coconut oil. Coconut oil is an antibacterial moisturizer—and it smells amazing. Add in some moisturizing honey and your skin will enjoy a beautiful, healthy, natural glow! Mix together the warmed coconut oil and honey. Soak a dry sheet mask in the liquid and apply to face. Leave on for 15 minutes and either pat remaining fluid into skin or wash face as usual.

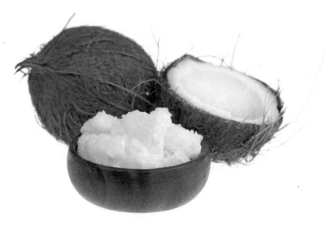

LEMON-LIME PHOTO-DAMAGE FIX MASK

1 tablespoon aloe vera gel
1 tablespoon lemon juice
1 tablespoon lime juice

Brighten the face and even out skin tone with this lemon-lime combo. This is best used at night, which allows your skin to recover before being exposed to the sun, as lemon and lime can increase skin sensitivity to it. Combine the ingredients and soak the dry mask. Apply the mask to your face and let sit for 15 minutes. Remove and pat the remaining fluid into the skin. Remember to follow up with sunscreen the next morning.

Lemon and lime juices can cause photosensitivity, so be sure to use them sparingly and to limit your skin's sun exposure after using them.

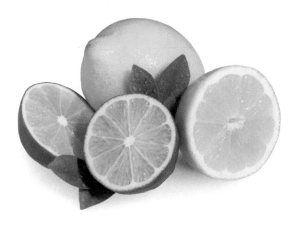

SPOTS-BE-GONE SKIN REPAIR MASK

2 egg whites
1 tablespoon lemon juice
1 tablespoon turmeric

This mask is perfect for treating scars, age spots, and sun damage. The egg whites and lemon juice brighten skin while the turmeric both brightens and repairs surface skin damage. For best results use twice a week. Combine the ingredients and soak a cotton sheet mask in the liquid. Apply mask to face and leave on for 15 minutes. Remove mask and rinse skin with warm water.

- -

Lemon juice can cause photosensitivity, so be sure to use it sparingly and to limit your skin's sun exposure after using it. Note that the turmeric will likely stain your sheet mask. So be prepared for this outcome or skip the sheet mask and apply the ingredients directly to the face. See page 21 for more info on the best way to handle turmeric.

- -

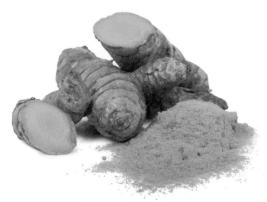

ROSE SPA SERUM MASK

2 tablespoons rose water
1 teaspoon rose hip seed oil
1 tablespoon aloe vera gel

Double up on the benefits of rose essence with this rose water
and rose hip seed oil mask. Combine the three ingredients.
Soak the dry sheet mask in the serum and apply mask to face.
Let sit for 15 minutes, then remove sheet mask, patting any
extra serum into the skin.

You can substitute any of your favorite face oils for rose hip seed oil.

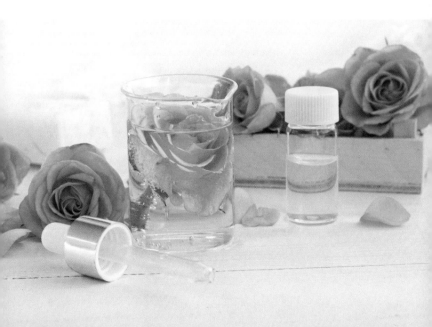

SUNBURN SERUM MASK

2 tablespoons aloe vera gel
1 tablespoon chamomile tea, cooled
1 teaspoon matcha powder
¼ avocado, mashed

Sunburns happen—even when we're careful to apply sunscreen. If you've accidentally fried your skin and need some relief, look no farther than the Sunburn Serum Mask that uses gentle, soothing aloe vera and chamomile to relieve the pain, and matcha powder and avocado to protect against and repair the UV damage. Combine the ingredients and soak the mask in the serum. Apply mask to face and let sit for 15 minutes. Remove mask and rinse gently with warm water.

- -

You can use finely ground green tea if you don't have matcha on hand.

- -

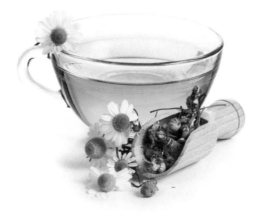

UNICORN SPARKLE SHEET MASK

2 tablespoons aloe vera gel
1 or 2 drops of red or blue food coloring
1 teaspoon multicolored glitter

This is a fun mask for birthday parties and any other time
you need a silly break from the seriousness of life. Add the
food coloring to the aloe and mix. Dip the mask in the liquid
until soaked through. Gently place the mask on a damp wash-

cloth or towel. Apply a sprinkle of glitter to the outside of
the mask. Carefully place the mask on the face, glitter side
out. Take a bunch of photos! When removing the mask, lift it
carefully from the face, ensuring all the glitter stays on the
mask. Rinse face carefully.

If you add too much food coloring
it may stain the skin, so be sure
to use just enough to lightly color
the aloe and the mask. You can
also make your own food coloring
using actual foods, like beets,
blueberries, and more. A
quick search online will
give you tons of options.

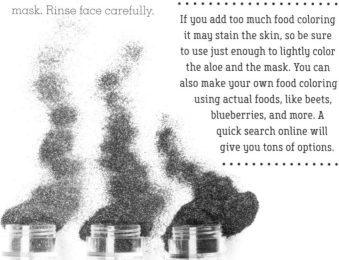

CLARIFYING & CLEANSING
SHEET MASKS

LIME + GRAPEFRUIT CITRUS BRIGHT MASK

1 tablespoon lime juice
1 tablespoon grapefruit juice

Lime and grapefruit have clarifying and astringent properties while also being packed with skin-tone-perfecting vitamin C. This is best used at night, which allows your skin to recover before being exposed to the sun. Combine the lime and grapefruit juices and then soak the dry mask in the liquid. Apply the mask to your face and let sit for 15 minutes. Pat the remaining fluid into the skin. Remember to follow up with sunscreen the next morning.

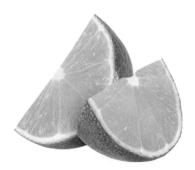

Lime and grapefruit juices can cause photosensitivity, so be sure to use it sparingly and to limit your skin's sun exposure after using it.

CLARIFYING MATCHA MASK

1 teaspoon matcha powder
2 tablespoons aloe vera gel

This simple two-ingredient mask uses antioxidant-packed matcha to help improve skin elasticity and to reduce inflammation, while the base is soothing, antibacterial aloe vera. Combine both ingredients and soak the cotton mask until saturated. Apply to face for 15 minutes. Rinse face in warm water.

- -

You can use finely ground green tea if you don't have matcha on hand.

- -

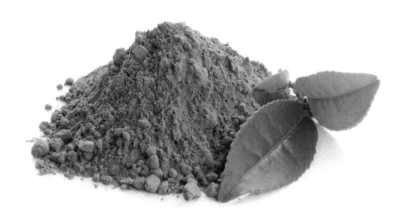

CLARIFYING &
CLEANSING

APPLE ACID EXFOLIATION MASK

1 teaspoon baking soda
2 tablespoons warm water
1 tablespoon apple cider vinegar
1 teaspoon honey

This is a powerful mask that provides natural, chemical exfoliation from malic acid along with a healthy dab of honey to calm and hydrate skin. Combine the ingredients (the baking soda will fizz when combined with the water and vinegar). Dip the dry sheet mask in the mixture and apply to face. Leave on for 5–10 minutes and gently rinse face with warm water.

· ·

This mask isn't recommended for sensitive skin due
to the extra exfoliation provided by the baking soda and
vinegar combo. Even if you don't have sensitive skin,
use this mask no more than once a week.

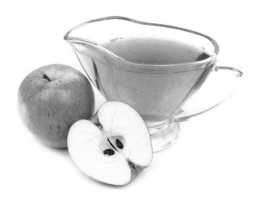

*"Wrinkles should merely indicate
where smiles have been."*
– Mark Twain

ACTIVATED CHARCOAL PURITY MASK

1 tablespoon activated charcoal
2 tablespoons whole milk

Activated charcoal is thought to draw out toxins and impurities in the skin, while the lactic acid in milk gently exfoliates. After application, this mask will help skin look clearer and feel softer. Combine the charcoal powder and milk. Dip the dry sheet mask in the liquid and apply to face. Leave on for 15 minutes, then wash face with warm water and a mild cleanser.

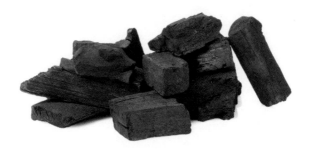

HONEY MOISTURE INTENSIVE
LIP MASK

1 teaspoon plain yogurt
1 teaspoon honey

Lip masks have become popular for their ability to deliver intense hydration that you just can't get from a lip balm. Let the lactic acid in the yogurt gently exfoliate your lips while the honey acts as a humectant to provide sweet moisture. Combine the yogurt and honey and then apply liberally to lips. Leave on for 5–10 minutes, then gently wipe off mask with a tissue.

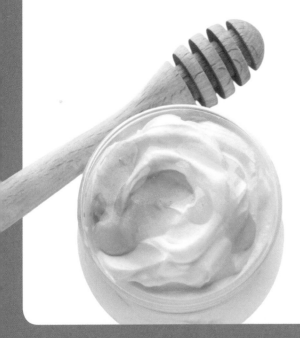

TONING & ACNE-FIGHTING
SHEET MASKS

EGG WHITE TIGHT-AND-BRIGHT MASK

2 egg whites
½ teaspoon turmeric powder

Egg whites work to tighten pores while turmeric can brighten your skin tone. This mask will leave your skin feeling tighter and smoother while giving you a healthy glow. Whisk the egg whites and turmeric together. Soak a cotton mask in the liquid and apply to your face for 15 minutes or until dry, then wash your face as usual.

Note that the turmeric will likely stain your sheet mask. So be prepared for this outcome or skip the sheet mask and apply the ingredients directly to the face. See page 21 for more info on the best way to handle turmeric.

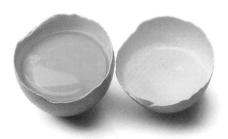

TURMERIC ANTI-ACNE MASK

2 tablespoons coconut oil, warmed
1 teaspoon honey
2 tablespoons turmeric

The antibacterial properties of coconut oil and honey with the antimicrobial and anti-inflammatory properties of turmeric make this a perfect mask for treating and controlling acne. Coconut also helps to control oil and to restore balance to acne-prone skin. Combine the ingredients and soak the mask in the liquid. Apply to face and let sit for 15 minutes. Remove mask and gently wash as usual.

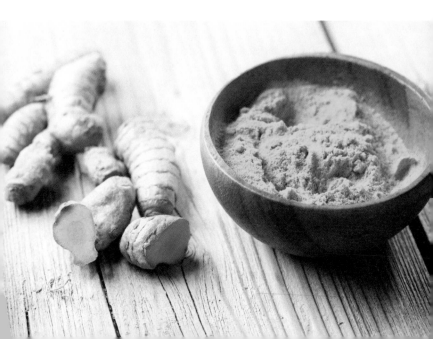

TEA TREE + LIME ACNE MASK

1–2 drops tea tree oil
2 tablespoons aloe vera gel
1 teaspoon lime juice
1 teaspoon water

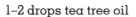

Clarifying tea tree oil combats acne alongside oil-controlling lime juice for a beat-the-spots mask that's great for once-a-week use. Combine the four ingredients and soak the dry sheet mask in the liquid. Apply sheet mask to face and leave on for 15 minutes. Remove mask and pat remaining liquid into skin.

• •

Lime juice can cause photosensitivity, so be sure to use it sparingly and to limit your skin's sun exposure after using it.

• •

**TONING &
ACNE-FIGHTING**

LIME + COCONUT ACNE MASK

2 tablespoons lime juice
1 teaspoon coconut oil, warmed

Lime juice is a great spot treatment for acne, and this mask goes one step further by targeting the whole face. The coconut oil acts to keep the lime juice from being too acidic and harsh on your face. Combine the lime juice and the coconut oil. Soak the mask in the mixture and apply to face. Leave on for 15 minutes, then remove and pat any remaining liquid into the skin. This is best used at night, which allows your skin to recover before being exposed to the sun. Remember to follow up with sunscreen the next morning.

- -

Lime juice can cause photosensitivity, so be sure to use it sparingly
and to limit your skin's sun exposure after using it.

- -

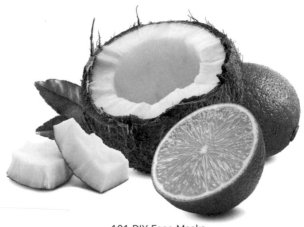

SIMPLE CIDER MASK

¼ cup warm water
2 tablespoons apple cider vinegar

This straightforward apple cider vinegar mask will leave your skin feeling soft, toned, and moisturized. Combine the water and vinegar. Dip the mask in the liquid and apply to face, leaving it until dry. Remove sheet mask and rinse face with warm water.

Don't use this mask more than once a week, as the apple cider vinegar can dry out your skin.

APPLES TO APPLES MASK

1 tablespoon apple cider
1 tablespoon apple cider vinegar

Vitamin C and AHAs are the key ingredients to this double-apple mask. Combine the cider and the vinegar and then dip a dry sheet mask into the liquid. Apply mask to skin and let sit for 15–20 minutes. Remove mask and pat remaining liquid into skin with your fingertips.

TURMERIC + LEMON-LIME MASK

1 teaspoon turmeric
1 tablespoon lemon juice
1 tablespoon lime juice

Toning and brightening skin is easy with the astringent citrus duo of lemon and lime. Add the skin-brightening turmeric to the lemon and lime juices and stir until dissolved. Soak the sheet mask in the citrus-turmeric liquid and apply to face for 15 minutes. Remove and wash with a gentle cleanser and water.

Lemon and lime juices can cause photosensitivity, so be sure to use them sparingly and to limit your skin's sun exposure after using them. Note that the turmeric will likely stain your sheet mask. So be prepared for this outcome or skip the sheet mask and apply the ingredients directly to the face. See page 21 for more info on the best way to handle turmeric.

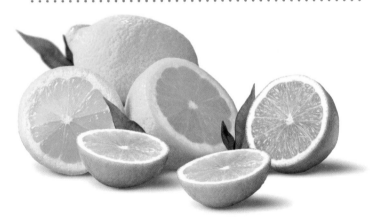

JACK-O'-LANTERN MASK

2 tablespoons canned pumpkin, mashed
2 tablespoons whole milk

Create your own special sheet mask just for Halloween. Using a pair of scissors and a new sheet of cotton, carefully design your own jack-o'-lantern sheet mask by cutting out fun mouth and eye holes. The spookier or sillier the better! Then combine the mashed pumpkin and milk until they form a paste and dip the spooky sheet mask into the liquid. Apply to face and leave on for 15 minutes. Rinse off remaining liquid and wash with a mild cleanser and water.

KID SAFE! This, and most of the masks in this book, are generally safe for children to use under supervision, if you are sure that none of the children are allergic to any of the ingredients and none of them are using any topical medicaiton. For children's parties, I like setting up "mask stations" with the individual dry sheet masks and ingredients set out in premeasured bowls in front of each placemat (or for older kids, the ingredients can be set out in big family-style bowls so they can measure themselves).

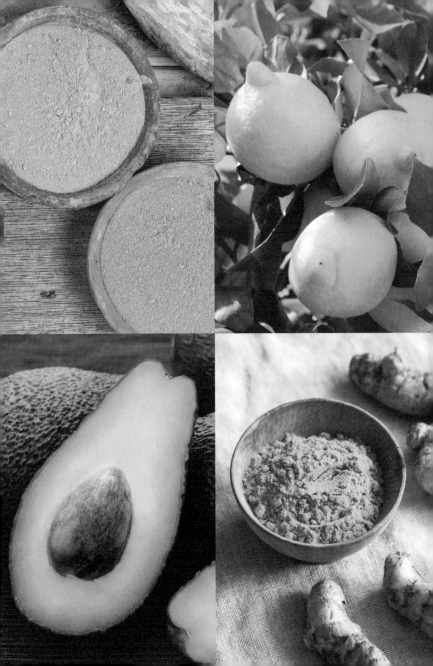

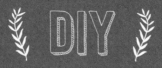

TRADITIONAL MASKS

"Glamour is about feeling good in your own skin."
– Zoë Saldana

The classic version of the face mask means the ingredients go from the fridge to your face—with no sheet mask in between! Get messy with ingredients like mashed pumpkin, banana, and avocado, or get exfoliating with an ingredient like brown sugar. There are masks here for every skin type, so experiment and see which one works best for you!

In general, ripe and even overripe fruit works best for face masks. You want soft ingredients as those are the best for your face. So avoid those rock-hard avocados! Many of the masks require just a small amount of fruit (a teaspoon of fresh lemon juice means a lot of lemon left over, for example); be sure to use the excess so nothing goes to waste. I recommend adding leftover ingredients to a smoothie. Or use watermelon, lemon, or lime slices as garnishes for cocktails!

SOOTHING & SOFTENING

TRADITIONAL MASKS

OATMEAL + CREAM SOFT SOOTHING MASK

2 tablespoons colloidal oatmeal
2 tablespoons heavy cream

This mask harnesses the soothing power of oatmeal and rich cream. It works well on dry, irritated, patchy skin that needs a bit of tender loving care. Combine the oatmeal and cream until well blended and then smooth over face and neck. Let sit for 15 minutes and rinse off with warm water.

PUMPKIN + OATMEAL EVERYDAY MASK

2 tablespoons canned pumpkin, mashed
1 tablespoon colloidal oatmeal

This mask is great for everyday use. The pumpkin and oatmeal treat skin gently while leaving it brighter and softer. Combine the ingredients and slather on the face and neck. Leave on for 15 minutes and remove gently with warm water.

MULTIPURPOSE CALMING MASK

1 tablespoon colloidal oatmeal
1 tablespoon hot water
1 teaspoon plain yogurt
1 teaspoon honey
1 egg white
1 teaspoon rose water

This soothing mask is perfect for sensitive and dry skin—slather it on and enjoy the heavenly feeling of nature's most effective calming ingredients. Mix oatmeal and hot water until combined. Stir in yogurt, honey, rose water, and egg white. Apply to face and neck and leave on for 15 minutes. Rinse off mask with warm water.

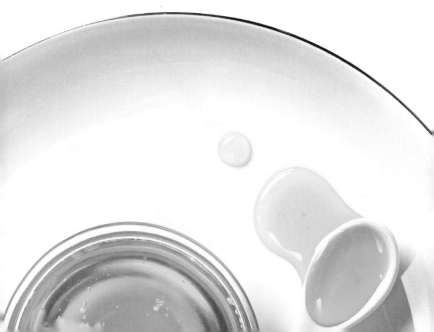

ENHANCED SEAWEED SPA FACIAL

2 strips dried seaweed, crushed
1 teaspoon aloe vera gel
1 teaspoon honey

Seaweed facials are commonly offered in expensive spas, but luckily you can replicate the results for a fraction of the cost. This is a soothing mask that will calm and treat skin while infusing it with minerals and vitamins. Add the aloe and honey to the crushed seaweed and combine until they form a paste. Slather mask onto face and neck and let sit for 15 minutes. Remove with warm water.

Make sure you get seaweed that doesn't have any additional ingredients, such as salt.

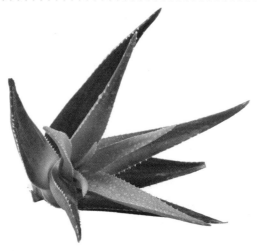

SEAWEED QUEEN OR
SEA CREATURE SHEET MASK

1 package of dried seaweed
2 tablespoons aloe vera gel
1 teaspoon multicolored glitter

Whether you want to be a scary sea creature from the deep or
a glistening seaweed queen, this is the mask for you. Nourishing seaweed and gentle aloe vera are great and everything—
but the fun comes from putting these glittery, green, slimy strips
of seaweed on your face!

Dip the seaweed strips in aloe until moist. Then gently lay
the seaweed on a damp washcloth or towel. Apply a sprinkle
of glitter to the outside of the strips. Carefully place the strips
on the face, glitter side out. Repeat until face and neck are
covered. Take a bunch of photos! When removing the mask, lift
each strip carefully from the face, ensuring all the glitter stays
on the strip. Rinse face carefully.

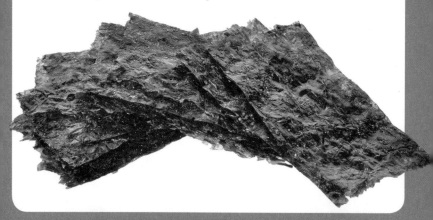

*"Beauty is about being comfortable
in your own skin. It's about knowing
and accepting who you are."*
– Ellen DeGeneres

BANANA + CHAMOMILE SOOTHING MASK

½ banana, mashed
2 tablespoons chamomile tea, cooled
1 teaspoon honey

When your skin has had enough and you're looking for something to calm and soothe it after a hard day, this is a great go-to mask. Nonirritating ingredients relax and repair your skin so you can face the world again. Combine the banana, chamomile, and honey together until well mixed. Apply mixture to face and leave on for 15 minutes. Rinse off with warm water.

BANANA BOAT VACATION MASK

½ banana, mashed
1 tablespoon coconut oil, warmed

You know those days when you just really want to inhale the breezy, beautiful scent of the ocean air? Or better yet, drink one of those fruity cocktails you get at the beach? Well you're in luck! The banana boat mask is basically a free vacation. Combine the banana and coconut oil and apply to face and neck. Let sit for 15 minutes. Sip a piña colada through a straw while the mask works its magic. Rinse with warm water.

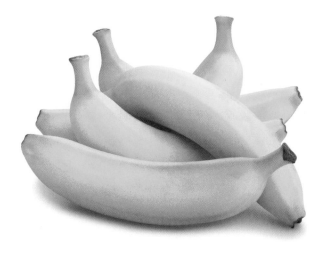

CALMING COLLOIDAL OATMEAL + CLAY MASK

1 teaspoon bentonite clay
1 teaspoon colloidal oatmeal
1 teaspoon rose water

These calming ingredients combine to create a powerhouse mask. This will soothe your tired, dull skin, and reduce redness without drying out your skin. Combine clay, oatmeal, and rose water to form a paste. Apply to face and neck and leave on for 15 minutes. Rinse with warm water.

PINK CLAY, OATMEAL + ALOE MASK

2 tablespoons French pink clay
1 tablespoon aloe vera gel
1 teaspoon colloidal oatmeal
1 teaspoon water

A soothing, clarifying mask for sensitive or dry skin. Combine the clay, aloe, oatmeal, and water to form a paste. Smooth over dry skin and leave on for 15 minutes. Remove with warm water.

HYDRATING & NOURISHING
TRADITIONAL MASKS

MATCHA, MILK + BANANA MASK

½ banana, mashed
1 tablespoon matcha powder
1 tablespoon whole milk

Nourishing, effective, and easy to make, this milky mask delivers moisture and nutrients for healthy, glowing skin. Combine the ingredients and slather onto face and neck. Let dry for 15 minutes and rinse off gently with warm water.

• •

You can use finely ground green tea if you don't have matcha on hand.

• •

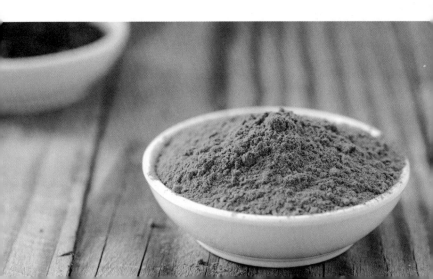

SEAWEED-POWER MINERAL MASK

1 tablespoon French green clay
1 tablespoon aloe vera gel
2 strips dried seaweed, crushed

Green clay gets its color from ancient seaweed, which means the clay is packed with minerals and vitamins that deliver great results for your skin. This mask doubles the seaweed quotient for extra powerful plant-based nourishment. Combine the clay, aloe, and seaweed and then apply to face and neck. Let dry for 15 minutes, then wash off with warm water and a gentle cleanser.

. . . .

Make sure you get seaweed that doesn't have any
additional ingredients, such as salt.

. . . .

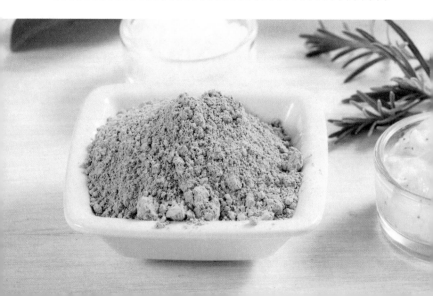

BANANA + COCONUT MOISTURE MASK

½ banana, mashed
1 tablespoon coconut oil, warmed

Protein-packed banana with healing and moisturizing coconut combine to give you a hydrated and nourished feeling. Mash the banana with the back of a fork and add the coconut oil until combined. Apply to face and let sit for 15 minutes. Rinse off with warm water.

FLAKE-REPAIR BANANA MASK

½ banana, mashed
2 tablespoons aloe vera gel
1 teaspoon honey

Dry skin can be tough to get a handle on—especially dry, flaky skin that doesn't seem to hold moisture no matter how hard you try. Combine the three ingredients and apply mask to face. Leave on for 15 minutes and gently rinse off with warm water.

BROWN SUGAR + COCONUT HYDRATE-AND-GLOW MASK

1 tablespoon brown sugar
1 tablespoon coconut oil, room temperature
1 teaspoon honey

Enjoy the exfoliating properties of sweet brown sugar while letting the hydrating coconut oil melt into your skin to provide hydration and a healthy glow. Mix the three ingredients together, applying in a circular motion to the face and neck. Leave on for 15 minutes and wash off using circular motions until the brown sugar is rinsed away.

. . . .

Brown sugar should be used no more than once a week, especially if you have sensitive skin. This mask is best used before bed to allow for overnight absorption of the coconut oil residue into the skin.

. . . .

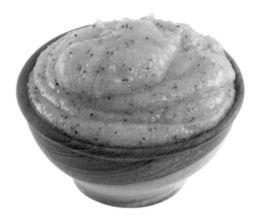

DAIRY MILK MASK

2 teaspoons cocoa powder
1 tablespoon whole milk
1 tablespoon buttermilk

Cocoa provides an antioxidant punch in this delicious smelling
(and tasting!) mask. The cocoa nourishes your skin and the milk
and buttermilk provide moisture and exfoliation. Combine the
three ingredients and apply to face. Leave on for 15 minutes and
rinse off with a gentle cleanser and warm water.

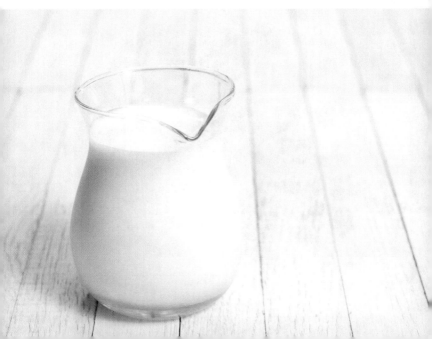

COCOA REPAIR +
REVEAL LIP MASK

1 teaspoon honey
1 teaspoon cocoa powder

Try not to lick your lips too hard (I know it's tough!) while the honey and cocoa soothe and repair dry, tired skin. Combine the two ingredients until they form a paste. Rub in a circular motion onto lips and let sit for 10 minutes. Gently wipe off any excess mask with a tissue.

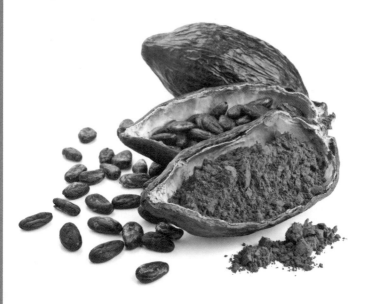

WATERMELON + BANANA INTENSE REPAIR MASK

¼ cup watermelon juice
½ banana, mashed

Watermelon delivers vitamins, nutrients, and a burst of hydration while the banana doubles up extra moisture and brightening. Add the watermelon juice to mashed banana until combined. Spread mixture over face and leave on for 20 minutes. Gently wash off with warm water.

AVOCADO MOISTURE INTENSIVE NIGHT MASK

½ avocado, mashed
1 teaspoon coconut oil, room temperature
1 teaspoon honey

This luxurious moisture mask is packed with hydration and will leave your skin supple and nourished. It's a great one to do before bed, so your skin can relax and absorb the extra moisture left behind by the coconut oil overnight. Mix the mashed avocado, coconut oil, and honey together and then spread mixture over face and neck. Leave on for 15 minutes. Rinse gently with warm water but no soap.

KIWI + AVOCADO MASK

½ avocado, mashed
½ kiwi, mashed
1 teaspoon honey

This high-hydration mask gives you the power of avocado and the brightening effect of kiwi with all of its vitamin C. Add in a dollop of honey as an antibacterial and moisturizing treat, and you've got a stellar mask for weekdays or weekends. Or every day! Combine the avocado, kiwi, and honey together and smooth over face and neck. Let sit for 15 minutes and rinse off with warm water.

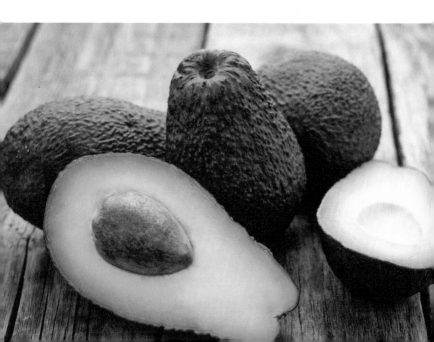

MILK MOISTURE MASK

1 tablespoon whole milk
1 tablespoon plain yogurt

Double your lactic acid application with this milky moisture mask. Combine the milk and yogurt together. Apply to face and neck and let sit for 15 minutes. Rinse off with warm water.

KIWI + BANANA FRESH MASK

½ kiwi, mashed
½ banana, mashed
1 teaspoon honey

Kiwi, banana, and honey make for a moisture mask that can't be beat. Combine the ingredients until they form a paste. Apply directly to skin and let sit for 15 minutes. Rinse gently with warm water.

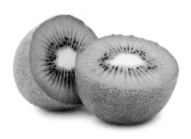

BRIGHTENING & REFRESHING

TRADITIONAL MASKS

RICE FLOUR + HONEY DAILY MASK

1 tablespoon rice flour
1 tablespoon honey

For correcting uneven skin tone and brightening dull skin, try this rice flour mask with a dollop of honey for moisture. Mix the rice flour and honey until a paste forms. Apply to skin and neck and let sit for 15 minutes. Rinse off with warm water.

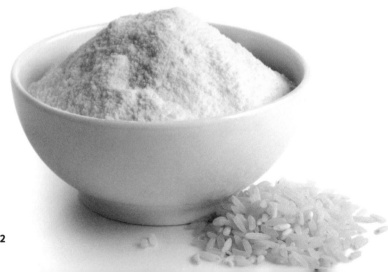

1 tablespoon rice flour

1 tablespoon whole milk

1 teaspoon turmeric

With lactic acid, ferulic acid, and curcumin all working to brighten skin, this is a highly effective mask that will leave your skin with a lovely glow. Combine the three ingredients until a paste forms. Smooth over face and neck. Leave on for 15 minutes and rinse with warm water and a gentle cleanser.

See page 21 for more info on the best way to handle turmeric.

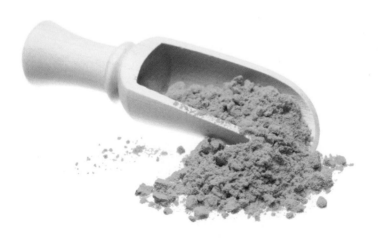

YOGURT + TURMERIC MOISTURE BRIGHTENING MASK

2 tablespoons plain yogurt
1 tablespoon turmeric

This is a great moisturizing, exfoliating, and brightening mask for dry and dull skin. Mix the yogurt and turmeric together and then smooth onto face and neck. Leave on for 15 minutes, then wash face as usual.

See page 21 for more info on the best way to handle turmeric.

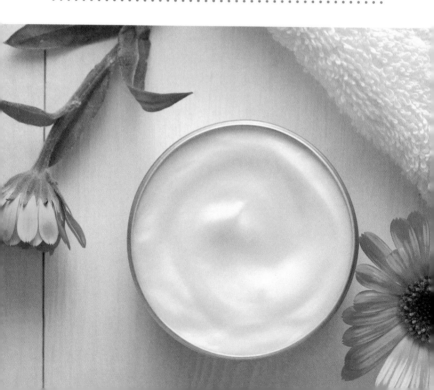

TURMERIC SKIN GLOW MASK

1 tablespoon turmeric
1 teaspoon coconut oil, warmed
2 tablespoons honey

Achieving healthy, natural, and glowing skin is the holy grail of skincare. Luckily, there's a natural, effective, and affordable way to get that glam glow! Turmeric along with coconut oil and honey combine to create a luxurious treatment for dry and dull skin. Combine ingredients together and apply to face and neck. After 15 minutes, rinse off mask with warm water and a gentle cleanser.

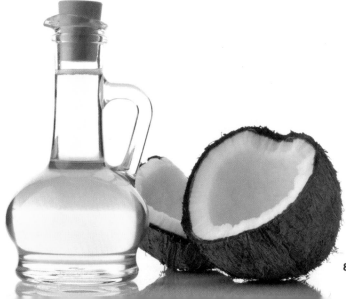

INTENSE BRIGHTENING TURMERIC + CLAY MASK

1 tablespoon turmeric
2 tablespoons bentonite clay
1 tablespoon water

Turmeric is a great tool for brightening skin and for combating age spots, acne scars, and other hyperpigmentation. This mask ups the power of turmeric by pairing it with bentonite clay—letting this high-powered mask penetrate the pores and brighten the skin at the same time. Combine the ingredients and apply to skin. Let dry completely and rinse off with a gentle cleanser and warm water.

See page 21 for more info on the best way to handle turmeric.

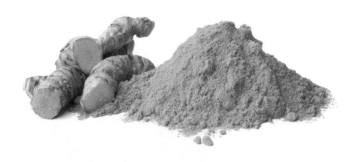

UNDERARM DETOX CARE MASK

1 tablespoon bentonite clay
1 tablespoon apple cider vinegar
1 teaspoon coconut oil, warmed
1 teaspoon lemon juice

Yep—your underarms need some love too! This mask is perfect for taking care of your pits that can get gunked up or dried out from daily deodorant use or irritated from shaving. Let the clay draw out impurities while the vinegar lightly balances the skin's pH levels. The coconut oil and lemon also team up to provide antibacterial protection. Combine the ingredients together and apply to underarm area. Leave on for 15 minutes, then rinse off (ideally in the shower to avoid a mess) and pat underarms dry with a towel.

Don't use this mask more than once a week, as the apple cider vinegar can dry out your skin.

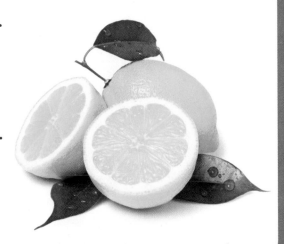

BRIGHTENING CIDER + PUMPKIN ENZYME MASK

¼ cup canned pumpkin, mashed
2 tablespoons apple cider vinegar
1 teaspoon water

Can you say, smells like autumn? This pumpkin and apple cider mask is good enough to eat. The pumpkin and cider vinegar combo helps brighten and tone skin while also controlling oil. Combine the pumpkin, water, and cider vinegar and then apply to face; leave on for 15 minutes. Rinse off with warm water.

Don't use this mask more than once a week, as the apple cider vinegar can dry out your skin.

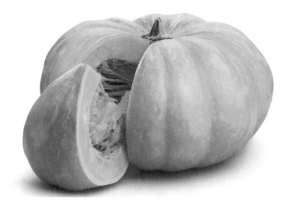

PUMPKIN SPICE LATTE MORNING MASK

1 tablespoon canned pumpkin, mashed
1 teaspoon finely ground coffee
1 teaspoon brown sugar
1 tablespoon whole milk

Get your pumpkin spice latte fix any time of year with this wake-up-my-face mask. The pumpkin works to brighten and firm up the skin, the coffee constricts blood vessels and reduces puffiness and redness, the brown sugar exfoliates, and the milk calms and treats inflammation. Talk about a mask that can do it all! Combine the ingredients and slather on the face and neck. Leave on for 15 minutes and remove gently with warm water.

. . . .
Brown sugar should
be used no more
than once a week,
especially if you have
sensitive skin.
. . . .

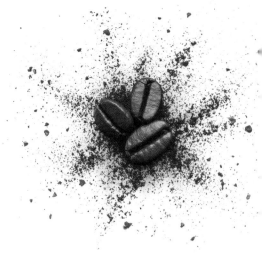

MILKY BROWN SUGAR REFRESH MASK

2 tablespoons brown sugar
2 tablespoons whole milk

The sugar crystals provide a gentle physical exfoliation while the lactic acid in the milk provides a light chemical exfoliation. As a bonus, the calming and moisturizing properties of the milk let you present a fresh, clean face to the world. Combine the sugar and milk and then gently apply to face in circular motions, avoiding the delicate under-eye area. Let dry for 15 minutes and rinse using circular motions until all the sugar is dissolved and your face is clean.

Brown sugar should be used no more than once
a week, especially if you have sensitive skin.

RICE FLOUR + YOGURT EXFOLIATION MASK

1 tablespoon rice flour
1 tablespoon plain yogurt

For brightening skin tone and gentle exfoliation, there's nothing better than soft rice flour and lactic acid. Mix the rice flour and yogurt until a paste forms. Apply to skin and neck and let sit for 15 minutes. Rinse with warm water.

RICE + CLAY BRIGHTEN-MY-DAY MASK

1 teaspoon rice flour

1 teaspoon lemon juice

1 teaspoon bentonite clay

1 teaspoon water

Rice flour and lemon juice are a powerful brightening duo while bentonite clay works to draw out impurities that make skin look dull. Together you'll find this mask works to maintain an even skin tone. Mix the flour, lemon juice, clay, and water together to form a paste. Apply to face and neck and leave on for 15–20 minutes. Rinse off with warm water.

- -

Lemon juice can cause photosensitivity, so be sure to use it sparingly and to limit your skin's sun exposure after using it.

- -

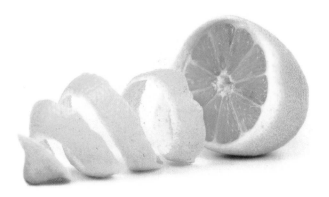

HEALING & ANTIAGING
TRADITIONAL MASKS

YOUTHFUL YOGURT + CAFFEINE MASK

2 tablespoons plain yogurt
1 tablespoon finely ground coffee
1 egg white

Yogurt gently chemically exfoliates while the caffeine and egg white tighten and tone skin for an overall healthy lift and youthful glow! Combine the ingredients and smooth over face and neck. Leave on for 15 minutes and rinse with a gentle cleanser and water.

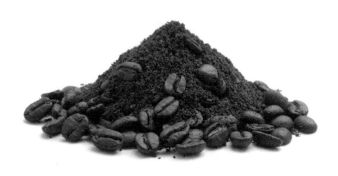

FLORAL RICE FLOUR MASK

1 tablespoon rice flour
1 teaspoon matcha powder
1 tablespoon rose water

Rice flour and matcha help to repair damaged skin. Combine the matcha, rice flour, and rose water to form a paste. Apply to face and neck and let sit for 15 minutes. Rinse off with warm water.

You can use finely ground green tea if you don't have matcha on hand.

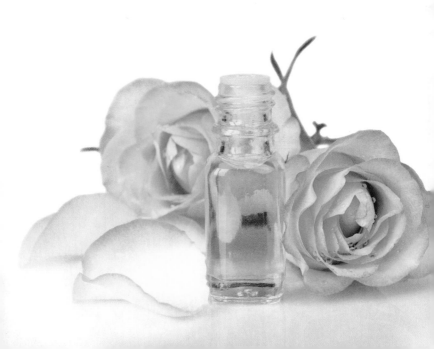

COLLAGEN EGG + ALOE MASK

1 egg white
2 tablespoons aloe vera gel

The egg white firms up the skin and tightens pores, while the aloe vera moisturizes to reduce lines and to nourish skin, making it look plumper. This is a great mask for refreshing aging or tired skin. Beat the egg white until frothy and add the aloe until combined. Smooth over face and neck and leave on for 15 minutes. Rinse gently with warm water.

SUPERFOOD CHOCOLATE + AVOCADO MASK

1 tablespoon cocoa powder
½ avocado, mashed

An infusion of collagen and antioxidants make this mask a great choice for aging skin or skin that needs a boost. Combine the cocoa powder and avocado to form a paste and apply to face. Leave on for 15 minutes and rinse off with a gentle cleanser and water.

ANTIOXIDANT-INFUSING MATCHA MASK

1 teaspoon matcha powder
1 tablespoon coconut oil, room temperature

With antioxidant, free-radical-fighting matcha powder combined with antibacterial coconut oil, this mask is a great all-purpose one for dry, dull, or aging skin. Mix the matcha powder and coconut oil together. Smooth over face, rubbing the mask into the face and neck until mostly absorbed and leave on for 15 minutes. Rinse with a gentle cleanser and water.

You can use finely ground green tea if you don't have matcha on hand.

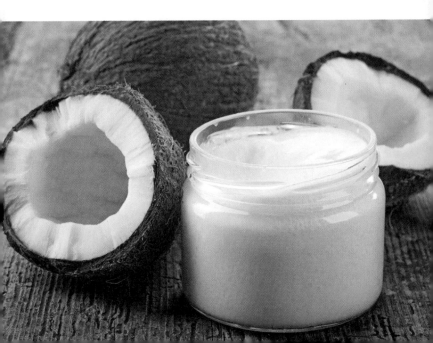

WICKED WITCH OF
THE WEST MASK

2 tablespoons French green clay
1 teaspoon matcha powder
2 tablespoons water
1 teaspoon finely ground coffee (optional)

Perfect for parties where you want to get a bit silly. Or treat yourself on Halloween and give those trick-or-treaters a fright! If you want to add a few warts and blemishes to complete your look, add a teaspoon of coffee grounds! Combine the ingredients and apply to face and neck. Leave on for 15 minutes (or for as long as you want your green look to last) and rinse off with a gentle cleanser and warm water.

. . . .

You can use finely ground green tea if you don't have matcha on hand.

. . . .

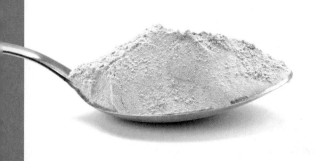

ROSE HIP SEED OIL + CLAY MASK

1 tablespoon bentonite clay
1 teaspoon rose hip seed oil
1 teaspoon honey

Exfoliate, repair, moisturize—this rose hip seed oil mask can do it all. Combine the clay, rose hip seed oil, and honey together to form a paste. Apply to face and neck and leave on for 15 minutes. Rinse off with warm water and enjoy the clean, soft feeling of your newly moisturized skin!

You can substitute any of your favorite face oils for rose hip seed oil.

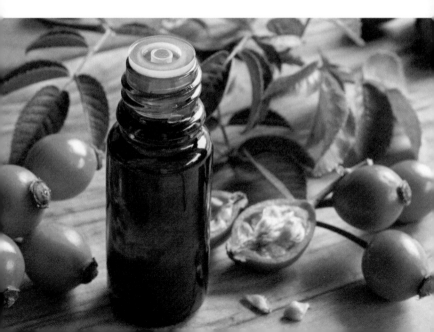

COCOA + LACTIC ACID MASK

1 tablespoon cocoa powder
1 tablespoon plain yogurt

Reduce the appearance of fine lines and puffiness with a caffeine and lactic acid mask. Combine the cocoa and yogurt until it looks like you're ready to make brownies. Smooth over face and neck and leave on for 15 minutes. Remove with warm water.

COFFEE + HONEY FIRMING MASK

1 tablespoon finely ground coffee
1 tablespoon honey

This is a simple mask for firming and revitalizing the skin. The caffeine acts to reduce redness and puffiness, while the honey plumps and hydrates. Combine the coffee and honey to form a paste and apply to face. Leave on for 15 minutes and rinse off with warm water.

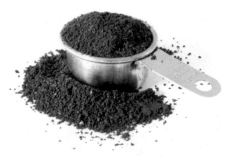

CLARIFYING & CLEANSING

DEEP CLEANSING BENTONITE CLAY MASK

1 tablespoon bentonite clay
1 tablespoon apple cider vinegar
1 teaspoon warm water

Bentonite clay is the ultimate deep cleanser. As the clay dries, it draws out impurities from the skin while the apple cider vinegar exfoliates and softens for a refreshed, natural glow. Mix the clay, apple cider vinegar, and water until they form a paste. Smooth over face and neck and let sit for 15 minutes or until mask is completely dry. Wash off with warm water.

· ·

Don't use this mask more than once a week, as the apple cider vinegar can dry out your skin.

· ·

CLAY + CHARCOAL PORE CLEANSING MASK

1 tablespoon bentonite clay
1 tablespoon activated charcoal
1 tablespoon water
1 teaspoon honey

Congested, clogged, and blackhead-prone skin? This is the mask for you. Allow the deep cleansing properties of the clay and activated charcoal to draw out impurities from your pores. Mix the ingredients together to form a paste and apply to face and neck. Leave on for 15 minutes or until completely dry, and wash with warm water and a gentle cleanser.

Your skin will feel a tingling sensation as this mask dries. Don't freak out—this is normal.

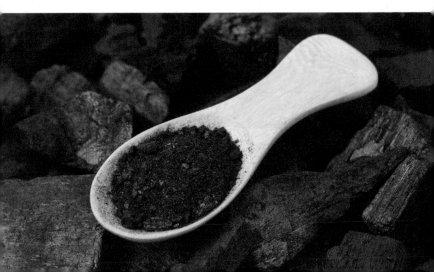

BLACKHEAD-BLASTING EGG WHITE MASK

2 egg whites
1 tablespoon lemon juice
1 teaspoon honey

The pore-tightening egg whites combined with the brightening properties of lemon juice will have your skin looking so fresh and so clean. Combine ingredients and spread over face. Let dry for 15 minutes. Rinse with warm water.

. . . .

Lemon juice can cause photosensitivity, so be sure to use it sparingly and to limit your skin's sun exposure after using it.

. . . .

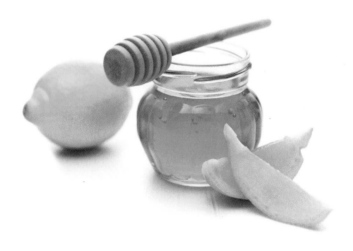

"The trick is to age honestly and gracefully and make it look great, so that everyone looks forward to it."

– Emma Thompson

CLEANSE-AND-REPAIR PINK CLAY + ALOE MASK

1 tablespoon French pink clay
1 teaspoon aloe vera gel
1 teaspoon coconut oil, warmed
1 teaspoon warm water

This gentle cleansing mask uses aloe vera gel and coconut oil to balance the potentially drying effects of the pink clay. This is great for anyone with dry or sensitive skin who wants to enjoy the deep cleansing benefits from the clay without the risk of skin that feels dehydrated afterward. Mix the pink clay, aloe vera gel, coconut oil, and water together until they form a paste. Apply mask to face and let dry for 15 minutes. Rinse off with warm water.

PINK WATERMELON + BROWN SUGAR EXFOLIATING MASK

2 tablespoons watermelon juice
1 tablespoon brown sugar

Light exfoliation and hydration make this a great mask for those sweaty and humid summer days when you just need to feel refreshed and bright. Combine the watermelon juice and brown sugar. Smooth mask over face and neck using circular motions until the mask is distributed evenly. Leave on for 15 minutes. Rinse off mask with warm water until the brown sugar is dissolved and skin is clean. For heavier exfoliation add a bit more brown sugar.

. . . .

Brown sugar should be used no more than once
a week, especially if you have sensitive skin.

. . . .

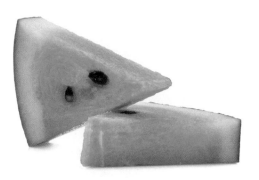

CLARIFYING & CLEANSING

PUMPKIN PATCH ENZYME MASK

1 egg white
¼ cup canned pumpkin, mashed
1 teaspoon honey

Take advantage of pumpkin's natural exfoliating abilities and slather on this mask packed with enzymes and natural acids. It will help your face appear smoother, firmer, and a bit more plump thanks to the collagen in the pumpkin. Froth the egg white and combine with the pumpkin and honey. Apply to face and leave on for 15 minutes. Rinse gently with warm water.

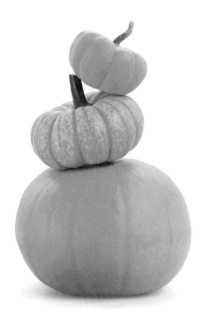

CHARCOAL PURIFYING AND CLARIFYING MASK

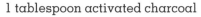

1 tablespoon activated charcoal
1 tablespoon apple cider vinegar
1 tablespoon honey
1 teaspoon water

Activated charcoal draws out impurities from the skin while the apple cider vinegar provides essential exfoliation. The honey is a sweet bonus to help calm and soothe the skin! Combine ingredients and apply to face. Leave on for 15 minutes and rinse with a gentle cleanser and warm water.

Don't use this mask more than once a week, as the apple cider vinegar can dry out your skin.

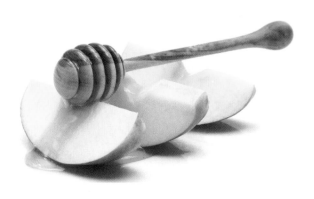

CHARCOAL + ALOE DETOX-SO-I-CAN-RETOX MASK

1 tablespoon activated charcoal
2 tablespoons aloe vera gel

The charcoal draws out impurities from the skin and lightly exfoliates, while the aloe vera cleanses, soothes, and boosts moisture levels—leaving skin cleansed, refreshed, and plumped. Mix ingredients together and smooth onto face and neck. Leave on for 15 minutes, then wash with a gentle cleanser and water.

THE CHOCOLATE FACIAL MASK

1 tablespoon cocoa powder
1 tablespoon honey

The antioxidant power of the cocoa plus the antibacterial and humectant powers of the honey make a potent (and delicious!) mask. Combine the cocoa powder and honey until they form a paste. Smooth over face and neck and leave on for 15 minutes. Remove with warm water and a gentle cleanser.

EGGS-TRAORDINARY PROTEIN
POWER HAIR MASK

2 egg whites
¼ cup plain yogurt

The protein found in both the eggs and the yogurt will help strengthen hair that's broken, damaged, or thinning. Froth the egg whites and combine with the yogurt. Apply the mask to dry hair, starting at the roots and working toward the ends. Leave on for 30 minutes and shampoo and condition as normal.

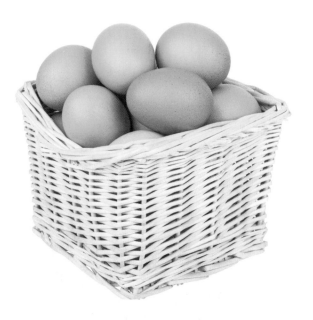

HONEY, BROWN SUGAR + LEMON SCRUB MASK

1 tablespoon lemon juice
1 tablespoon coconut oil, room temperature
1 tablespoon brown sugar

Lemon juice brightens the skin and acts as an astringent while the coconut oil acts as an antibacterial and moisturizer. Add in a dollop of brown sugar for gentle exfoliation and you have a great mask for all skin types. Combine the ingredients and apply to face with gentle circular motions. Let sit for 15 minutes and rinse off gently with warm water.

• •

Brown sugar should be used no more than once a week, especially if you have sensitive skin. Lemon juice can cause photosensitivity, so be sure to use it sparingly and to limit your skin's sun exposure after using it.

• •

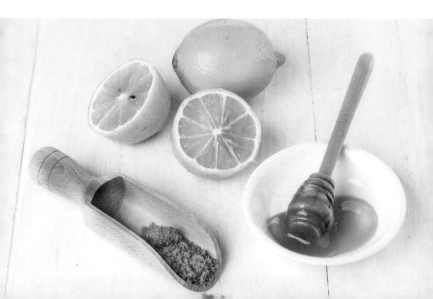

PINK ROSE MASK

1 tablespoon fresh pineapple juice
1 tablespoon French pink clay
1 tablespoon rose water

Draw out impurities and exfoliate with the power duo of pineapple and pink clay. A helping of rose water helps to soothe
the skin and keep it supple. Combine the pineapple, clay, and
rose water together and then apply to face and neck. Allow to
dry for 15 minutes and rinse off with warm water.

EXFOLIATION KIWI GLOW MASK

1 tablespoon plain yogurt
½ kiwi, mashed
1 tablespoon coconut oil, warmed

Lactic acid in the yogurt plus the vitamin C in the kiwi exfoliate the skin and repair sun damage while the coconut oil
moisturizes and maintains that skin glow we all love. Combine
the yogurt, kiwi, and coconut oil and then apply to face and
neck. Leave on for 15 minutes, then rinse off with warm water.

CLARIFYING & CLEANSING

SUGAR, LIME + HONEY SCRUB

1 tablespoon honey
1 tablespoon lime juice
1 teaspoon brown sugar

This fresh trio of ingredients offers a quick skin pick-me-up for anyone with dull skin. Combine the honey, lime, and brown sugar together and spread in circular motions over the face and neck. Leave on for 15 minutes, then rinse off gently with warm water and a gentle cleanser.

• •

Brown sugar should be used no more than once a week, especially if you have sensitive skin. Lime juice can cause photosensitivity, so be sure to use it sparingly and to limit your skin's sun exposure after using it.

• •

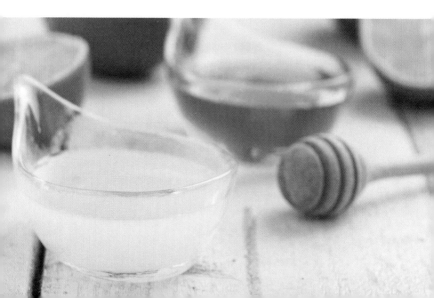

SUNRISE BRIDAL BLUSH MASK

1 tablespoon French pink clay
1 tablespoon rose water

Calling all brides and bridesmaids! When a simple deep clean just isn't enough, add a hint of pink blush to your skin-care routine with this nonirritating, gentle cleansing mask. Combine the blush-toned clay and scented rose water and then apply to face and neck. Leave mask on for 15 minutes. Snap some photos of you and your besties. Rinse with a gentle cleanser and warm water. Now you're ready for the big day!

KIWI + PINEAPPLE ASTRINGENT MASK

½ kiwi, mashed
1 tablespoon pineapple juice

Peel away dry, dead skin cells and reveal a bright, fresh face with the glycolic acid in this kiwi and pineapple astringent mask. Combine the kiwi pulp and the pineapple juice and apply to face and neck. Let sit for 15 minutes, then rinse off with warm water.

PINK PINEAPPLE MASK

1 tablespoon French pink clay
1 tablespoon pineapple juice

Fresh, pink, and pineapple! Your skin will look radiant after this detoxifying mask with the benefit of brightening pineapple enzymes. Combine the clay and pineapple until a paste forms. Apply to face and neck and leave on for 15–20 minutes. Rinse with warm water.

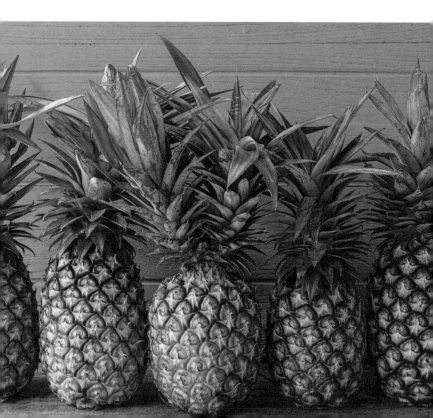

LACTIC ACID GREEN GIRL MASK

1 teaspoon matcha powder
1 teaspoon French green clay
1 tablespoon plain yogurt

For a light lactic acid treatment that also includes a detox plus antioxidant, this is your daily go-to. Mix the matcha, green clay, and yogurt together. Slather onto your face and neck and leave on for 15–20 minutes. Rinse with warm water to reveal clearer, brighter, and less congested skin.

You can use finely ground green tea if you don't have matcha on hand.

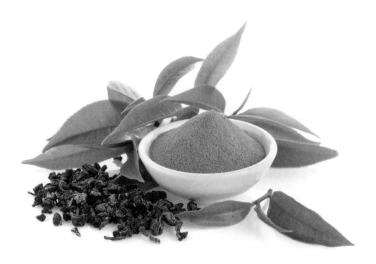

TONING & ACNE-FIGHTING
TRADITIONAL MASKS

ALL-PURPOSE DAILY OATMEAL MASK

1 tablespoon colloidal oatmeal
1 tablespoon honey
1 egg white

This gentle, multipurpose mask works to cleanse, firm, and exfoliate the skin. Combine ingredients and apply to face. Let dry for 15 minutes, then rinse with warm water. Use daily when you wake up or before you go to bed.

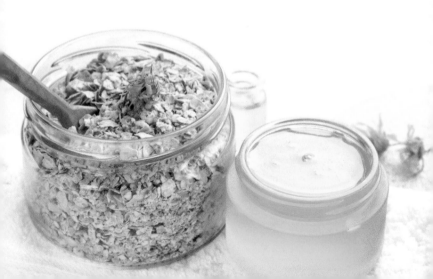

WAKE-ME-UP COFFEE UNDER-EYE MASK

1 egg white
1 tablespoon finely ground coffee

Egg whites tighten the skin while the caffeine in the coffee reduces swelling and puffiness. Beat the egg white until frothy and combine with the coffee grounds. Gently pat the mixture under the eye area. Leave on for 15 minutes and rinse off carefully with warm water.

> It's very important to ensure you're using finely ground, almost silty coffee here. Larger grounds can be too tough for the sensitive under-eye skin.

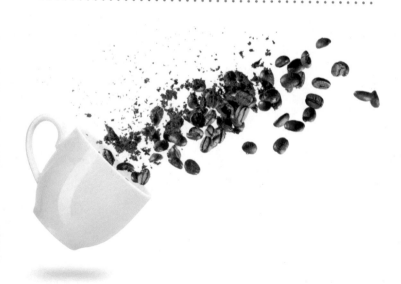

BLACKHEAD BLASTING SODA MASK

1 tablespoon baking soda
2 tablespoons coconut oil, warmed

Let the baking soda gently exfoliate and cleanse pores while the coconut oil acts as an antibacterial to keep skin clear. Combine the baking soda and coconut oil until they make a paste. Apply to face and leave on for 15 minutes. Gently rinse off with warm water.

· ·

Don't use baking soda too frequently or you could disrupt your skin's natural acidity. It's also not good for sensitive skin.

· ·

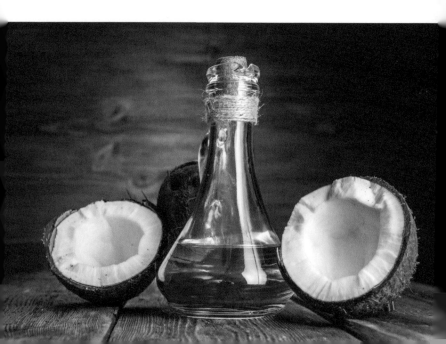

"How I feel about myself is more important than how I look. Feeling confident, being comfortable in your skin—that's what really makes you beautiful."

– Bobbi Brown

OIL CONTROL, LIGHT MOISTURE AVOCADO MASK

½ avocado, mashed
½ banana, mashed
1 egg white

The avocado and banana provide natural moisture that balances oily skin, while the egg white tightens the skin and controls extra oil production. Combine all the ingredients together and apply mask to face. Let dry for 15 minutes and rinse with warm water and a gentle cleanser.

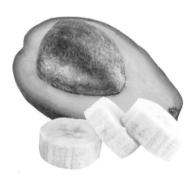

REVITALIZING SHINE MASK FOR DAMAGED HAIR

1 banana, mashed
1 tablespoon honey
¼ cup whole milk
1 egg white
1 tablespoon coconut oil, warmed

This is a great all-purpose mask for repairing dry and damaged hair. It also works well as a preventative mask to keep your hair looking healthy and shiny. Combine ingredients and slather mixture through dry hair, starting at the roots and working your way to the ends. Leave in for 1 hour. Wash hair with mild shampoo but don't use conditioner as the mask will act as your conditioner.

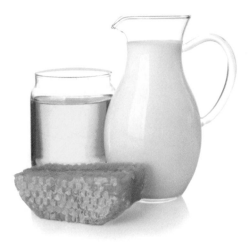

OLIVE OIL + KIWI MASK

1 teaspoon olive oil
½ kiwi, mashed
1 egg white

Nourishing, supple olive oil combined with toning kiwi and tightening egg white makes for a mask that plumps as it tightens. Mix the olive oil, kiwi, and egg white together. Apply to face and neck and leave on for 15 minutes. Rinse with warm water and a gentle cleanser.

ALOE ACNE MASK

1 tablespoon aloe vera gel
1 tablespoon honey

Soothing, healing aloe vera and antibacterial honey make for a simple and gentle mask for problem skin. Combine the ingredients and smooth over face and neck. Leave on for 15 minutes, then rinse gently with warm water.

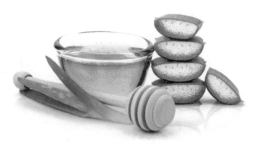

ROSE + TURMERIC MASK

1 teaspoon rose hip seed oil
1 teaspoon turmeric
1 teaspoon honey
1 tablespoon plain yogurt

Fight blemishes and signs of aging with a rose hip and turmeric lactic acid yogurt mask. Combine the rose hip seed oil,
turmeric, honey, and yogurt until well blended. Smooth over
face and neck and leave on for 15 minutes. Remove with warm
water and a gentle cleanser.

You can substitute any of your favorite face oils for rose hip seed oil.
See page 21 for more info on the best way to handle turmeric.

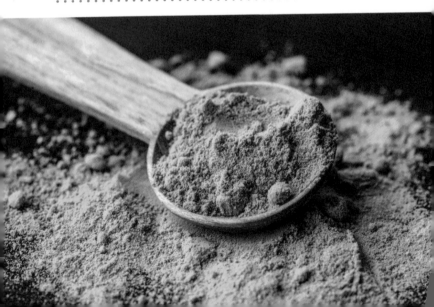

CAFFEINE LIFT MASK

1 tablespoon finely ground coffee
1 tablespoon cocoa powder
1 egg white
1 teaspoon water

Reduce inflammation and puffiness with caffeine while tightening pores with egg white. Combine coffee and cocoa powder with the egg white and water until smooth. Spread on face and neck and leave on for 15 minutes. Remove with warm water and a gentle cleanser.

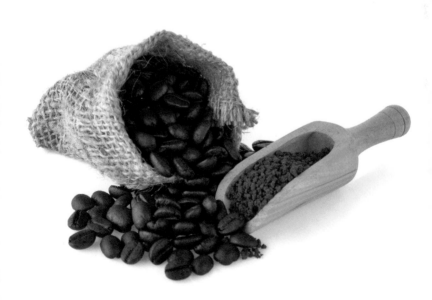

TONING & ACNE-FIGHTING

FRENCH GREEN CLAY + PINEAPPLE MASK

1 tablespoon pineapple juice
1 tablespoon French green clay

The pineapple (originally cultivated in South America) and French green clay (found in, you guessed it, France) combine here to create a fresh, healthy, impurity-fighting mask that targets skin imperfections and irregularities. Slather this on and enjoy softer skin—perfect for your upcoming vacation to São Paulo or Marseille. Combine the pineapple juice and clay until blended and slather onto face and neck. Let dry for 15 minutes, then wash off with a bit of a gentle cleanser and warm water.

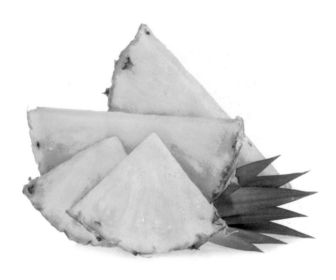

CHARCOAL + HONEY MASK

1 teaspoon activated charcoal
1 teaspoon honey
1 egg white

Honey, I shrunk my pores! The key to this pore reduction mask is the activated charcoal that draws out impurities and the skin-tightening properties of egg white. The honey is a soothing bonus that keeps skin hydrated and plump looking. Add the charcoal and honey to the egg white and mix until combined. Spread the mixture over your face and neck and let sit for 15–20 minutes. Rinse with warm water.

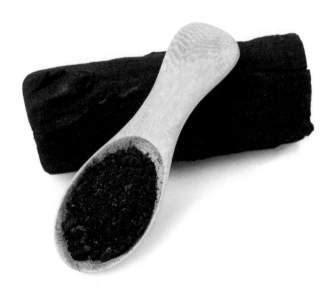

INDEX

For information about
special discounts for bulk
purchases, please contact
W. W. Norton Special
Sales at
specialsales@wwnorton
.com or 800-233-4830

Manufacturing by
Versa Press
Book design by Ashley
Prine, Tandem Books
Production manager:
Devon Zahn

The Countryman Press
www.countrymanpress
.com

A division of
W. W. Norton &
Company, Inc.
500 Fifth Avenue,
New York, NY 10110
www.wwnorton.com

978-1-68268-311-8 (pbk.)

10 9 8 7 6 5 4 3 2 1